The Ultimate 14-Day Candida Diet Cure

Candida Cure Recipes, Complete Guide To
Cleanse Your System, Cure Your Infection, And
Restore Health Fast

By Natalie Peterson

Copyright Information

Contents

Introduction

Hello, and thank you for taking the time to look at this book!

Candida is a major problem for some people. It's a way to really mess up your immune system, cause problems in the body, and leave you susceptible to immunological issues. Candida is never fun to combat, and often, not easy to combat. The candida diet, however can help you with your body.

What many don't realize is that our gut does need to have its own health maintained. If we don't do that, it can cause problems such as weight gain, mental health problems, and even major immune diseases that have trouble being combated. Candida is a problem that many of us don't even know about, because often, it's a problem at the bottom of many health concerns.

Often, when your doctor tells you that you have candida, you're probably worried about how to go about fixing it. The thing with candida is that it is hard to fix, but there are some ways to help with it. Although it does take time to combat this, you can bring your body back to the health that it had before, and the candida diet can help with this.

This book will go over what the candida diet is, some major parts of it, and even some recipes as well. The candida cure is also outlined in this as well, and you'll be able to get rid of it if you follow this for 90 days.

After 14 days on the candida diet, you'll be able to rectify the issues present within your gut, which is more than enough for many people.

Take the time to fix your health today though the candida diet, and you'll be able to make major changes that help your body out in many ways. By doing this, you'll be able to have the success you want, and the body you desire that is healthy and happy as well.

I used to suffer from candida. It was awful, and I had a multitude of factors that came about because of the fungus. However, once I took on the candida diet, I started to change my body for the better. I was healthier, happier, and I didn't have to worry as much about my gut health.

I wrote this book to help anyone with candida concerns and to give you a means to cure your candida so you can stop suffering from it.

Book Description

Do you know of the optimum and sure-fire way to beat candida?

Candida is a condition that can cause a lot of trouble for the body. From digestive issues to even immune system struggles, candida is not a fun illness to combat.

Fortunately, there is a way to beat this, and this book will show you just how to cure candida.

This book will go over the following information about candida:

- Why you must treat candida

- The candida cleanse

- The cure for candida

- What to eat and what not to eat

- Recipes to help combat symptoms

This book will show you what you need to know to bring you above and beyond your struggles that you may have with candida. You don't have to suffer any longer because this book will show you just how to combat the effects of candida through the use of dieting and eating healthy food.

CHAPTER 1

Why Treating Candida Is Important

Candida treatment is so very important. Candida is a major concern in many people, and it can cause a multitude of problems. This chapter will go over why treating candida is the most important part of candida treatment because it all starts with you.

With candida, most people don't catch it until it has gotten severe. The problem with candida is that it usually gets misdiagnosed, but if you don't catch it, it can wreak enormous damages to your immune and digestive systems.

Often, the big symptoms are the yeast infections one gets, the irritable bowel that many suffer from, and some of the headaches and itches. However, candida has a whole slew of symptoms, so it often doesn't get treated until it's too late.

Candida is a pathogen that causes a whole lot of trouble in your gut. Let's start with a bit of anatomy. Your gut has bacteria. These bacteria help you digest food and keep it cleaned out. However, let's say you get sick, and you take antibiotics.

These antibiotics not only kill the bad bacteria that is trying to get taken out, but it will take out the good bacteria in your gut as well. Stress and a diet full of sugar can cause this too, hence why diet is a major factor of this treatment.

Now, when the balance is not kept, candida spreads rapidly and will take over your gut. Candida is present within many people, but often, it's checked by the other bacteria in the body. However, this pathogen, when not stopped, causes a ton of different issues in the body.

Candida has 79 different byproducts including a neurotoxin called acetaldehyde and uric acid. The neurotoxin that is present causes headaches and brain fog. Recently, it was considered a carcinogen that can cause cancer. Uric acid causes arthritis and joint buildup. That's not even touching what the pathogen can cause in your gut.

Your gut is where most of the problems lay. If you suffer from candida, your gut will start to suffer from issues that can lead to an inability to effectively digest certain foods and issues with digestion, oral thrust, some yeast infections, food intolerances, and even allergies as well.

Candida is a type of bacteria that causes so many different problems. Many people might suffer from a multitude of symptoms before it gets handled.

Now, about 70% of us do have candida within us. However, most of the time it's under control, and the bacteria within your gut is the ruler over it. Candida becomes problematic in those who don't maintain the balance.

You probably have heard that doctors misconceive candida as something only a few that have a compromised immune system suffer from, such as those with AIDS, cancer, and other immune system disorders. Candida can be found in these types of patients, and it does have other issues that come along with that.

However, if you have a diet that is high in sugar and various antibiotics, then you're likely to develop this in your body as well. If you have a stressful life, then that adds more fuel to the fire. Nowadays, there is the candida antibiotics test that will tell you if you suffer from candida and if your body is working to fight it.

Now, when doctors speak of systemic candida, it typically means the candida that is seen in patients with severe illness and is life-threatening. Therefore, it needs to be monitored.

However, if you're suffering from candida and don't have that issue, then it's considered a candida overgrowth. This means that the candida infestation is happening in your gut for the most part. Often, you'll feel the symptoms that can be affecting you, such a recurring yeast infections, issues with digestion, and even headaches as well.

Candida can turn nasty if you're not careful. Often, people don't treat it until it's too late. They usually are told that it's an entirely different issue. You might be prescribed medicines that are helpful with the one symptom, but it doesn't tackle the whole issue.

The thing about candida is that if you are burdened with this disorder, then you'll never get rid of it unless you start to change something within your body. That's where this book comes in. It will go over what you need to do in order to help stop candida at its tracks and rectify the issues of candida over time.

CHAPTER 2

The Candida Cleanse

The first way to tackle candida is to do a cleanse. This is not only good for your gut, but will also help your liver, gallbladder, kidneys, and urinary system. If you're going to begin candida treatment, you should do so with a cleanse.

Now, with a candida cleanse, your target area is the colon because this is where many candida colonies are sitting around. It's a good place to begin when you're trying to do away with candida, and it will help reduce candida overgrowth. This is good for those who suffer moderate to severe cases of candida.

Now, when you're trying to do a candida cleanse, often people have a hard time keeping with it. When people cleanse, their energy levels are affected, and they might suffer from fatigue. With candida, it's already hard for them because when they do go through it, they might suffer from the low energy levels already. The cleanse just seems to add more fuel to the fire.

With the candida cleanse, it's advised that you eat a few small portions throughout the cleanse. You could be adventurous and do a full liquid diet, but if you are suffering too much, don't push yourself.

When you do this, you should follow the cleansing for 3-10 days if you want to do a full overhaul. If you're wanting to immediately lower your candida, you can do this and follow it for just the 3days.

What To Eat

The candida diet will be discussed later on in terms of what you should be eating, but this is basically a stricter version of the diet itself. Yes, candida already has a super strict diet.

Restricting it more will allow you to cleanse out your body quicker. So if you're looking to really get rid of the candida problem for good, then you will want to follow it. On this diet, you should focus mainly on having salads that are raw and veggies that are steamed.

You're probably looking at this and wondering how in the world you're going to do this. It only lasts for a few days which really isn't that bad.

For those who do it longer— like 7-10 days— it might be a bit tougher. However, your body will adjust after a couple of days. Soon, it'll make you feel refreshed, healthy, and even lighter in some cases.

Now, you should first take a moment to consider everything that you eat every single day prior to doing the candida cleanse. Often, you might not realize that your body is on overload, especially your liver and internal organs.

If you've been eating a lot of fast food, then you're probably overloading your body with unnecessary additives. If you eat a lot of beef, you're technically eating a ton of growth hormones too.

Even fish has chemicals from what is pushed into the oceans in their body. With oil companies spilling oil into the oceans from time to time, it's definitely wreaking havoc on your body.

Now, consider what will happen when you take the toxins out and replace them with veggies for the next few days. It will make a major change within you. If you suffer from candida, it will help in your fight against it.

With this cleanse, you should eat only salads that are raw and steamed veggies. Certain types of veggies should be avoided as well. Starchy veggies such as any type of potato, winter squash, yams, and even corn should be avoided because the starch will irritate the body during this cleanse.

Now, you probably don't really like the idea of a vegetable only diet. However, remember that you can flavor these with salt and pepper, various oils, some lemon juices, and include some spices and herbs to really liven it. It's not that hard. In truth, there is a lot that you can do with veggies for a few days.

If you're going to do the liquid-only cleanse, then you will need to make sure that you have extra nutrition. Often some vegetable broth is pretty good for this.

Vegetable broths are filled with nutrients, and you can use the liquid to help get the nutrients that you acquire from foods. You can use some vegetable broths that have veggies in it to give it flavor in order to help you go through with this cleanse.

If you're going to do the liquid-only cleanse, you will need to drink at least 2 or more bowls to really replace the minerals. Even if you're not doing the strict cleanse, a broth adds a little bit of flavor to your palate. You should use organic ingredients in order to help you get the full benefits.

For beverages, you should make sure you drink a ton of water. This will allow the body to clean itself up and flush out any toxins that might be present. The more water you drink, the better your body can work to eliminate toxins.

However, you should also think about some shakes. There are fiber shakes, bentonite shakes, and other sorts of liquids you can drink while on this diet. You should work to make sure you drink liquids that will support the liver, encourage bowel movements, and push the body to get rid of the candida toxins as quickly as possible.

If you are going to do this, make sure that you include as many toxins as possible. The types of shakes you can drink will be described in the recipe chapters later on.

Cleansing is much safer than you may think. It can help put your health back on track and get your liver functioning again in order to get rid of the toxins within your body.

However, this can be very stressful on the body. Therefore, if you suffer from major health problems, you should keep that in mind and let your doctor know before starting. If you start to have an irregular heartbeat or other symptoms that are cause for worry, you should make sure that you stop immediately for your safety.

It's also important to do this in a relaxed environment. If you're working a full-time job, you should try to get some time off. This is a health cleanse, so typically it's pretty easy to get the time that you need.

Keep your schedule free of any events, various commitments, and meetings. You can ideally do this during a weekend because it will only last a few days. However, if you need the full 10 days, don't be afraid to take it.

Cleansing is a great start for the candida diet, and it's very important that you do take this into consideration when focusing on treating candida. This chapter highlighted the cleanse you can start with to beat candida, so that you can really get the full benefits you need and stop candida in its tracks.

CHAPTER 3

An Outline Of The Candida Diet

The candida diet has a specific outline that can be used to help you really improve your body. Including these three elements will help you improve your candida diet, and it will allow you to help reverse the symptoms immediately.

Low Sugar Diet

The first thing to avoid is sugar. Now, candida needs organic carbon compounds to live and reproduce. The compounds switch it from a yeast to a fungal form. Sugars are what will help this thrive, so you need to cut out almost all sugars from your diet.

Now, often people think that they need to get rid of only added sugars for candida, but that is not the case. Natural sugars such as the ones in fruit will help the candida move right along and thrive just as well as soda.

If you're going to get rid of your candida, you're going to need to do away with the sugars entirely. This is pretty hard at first because often you might wonder how you're going to get rid of it all. In truth, many of the veggies that you have, along with some healthy meats and grains, can help you take out that dependence on sugar.

Now, the obvious foods such as any desserts, sugary snacks, various sodas that are riddled with sugar, and anything that has obvious sugar in it need to be avoided.

However, make sure to keep in mind that starchy veggies like potatoes and corn are also big-time culprits of this, and need to be treated the same as sugars in the first step of the diet. You will need to be diligent and read all food labels to allow you to cleanse out as many sugars as possible because food labels sneak those in like no other.

Now, you might feel anxious about what you can eat. In truth, there are a lot of great foods out there. You'll be able to eat non-starchy veggies, fish, some grains, and even meats to help bring together some great dishes. Herbs and spices will also liven up your food, and you won't have to worry about it being too hard on you.

Probiotics

With probiotics, often people think that they're just good bacteria. They are that, but they are necessary for this diet because this can be helpful with fighting off the candida and reducing the numbers.

Think about it; candida will struggle to thrive with a low-sugar diet. From there, the probiotics can step in and start to eat away at the candida before it worsens. You should have a probiotics period to help increase your gut health whether you have candida or not. You should also start to look at when you can add probiotics because often it does take a bit of cleansing before you can.

The probiotics will compete with the yeast that is created via candida within you. The nutrients are sparse, and with the reduction of sugar, the candida will have to work hard to even survive. That's where the probiotics come in.

They will do away with many of the candida yeast within the body. Often, it can be a good way to significantly reduce the fats. In addition, they will work to maintain the acidity within the stomach in a natural way.

Often, it will help to reduce the candida down to the bacteria and yeast that was harmless instead of a pathogenic fungus. Along with this too, the immune system will be boosted.

Often, you can get probiotics in various supplemental forms, and that's usually the best way to go about it. You can also get various fermented foods such as kefir and kimchi to help you get these good bacteria.

You should make sure that they are live cultures. Consult the labels for confirmation. You can also make your own probiotics at home if you're so pressed to have it as organic as possible, but it does take a bit of time.

Antifungals

Finally, there are antifungals. This is something that is either natural or prescribed by a doctor. You shouldn't introduce antifungals until the last third of the treatment because they often won't reverse candida outgrowth all on their own. However, if you combine this with the other two, it will help.

Often, people might get nystatin or another natural fungal, and people sometimes wonder if they should use the one prescribed or the natural one. Most of the time, the natural antifungals have fewer side effects, and you might need to take more to help get the same effect.

You don't rotate them because it gives the candida time to adapt. Therefore, if you're going natural, then just use all three at once. With a prescribed antifungal, they are typically stronger than the natural ones. The side effects can be straining on the body, so you should keep that in mind before you choose which one to get.

If you're looking for the right antifungal, you have a few options. Caprylic acid is an antifungal that's found in coconut oil, and it has antifungal properties that have been the subject of studies.

Oregano oil is a great fungi static and a fungicidal for the treatment of candida. It can help with other fungal pathogens as well. Grapefruit seed extract is also effective against at least 800 various bacterial and viral strains, and over 100 strains of fungi. It can also help with many other parasites as well. Often, people can use it and get significant results.

You can also get these antifungals on shelves at the store as well. If you want, garlic, olive oil, coconut oil, and also rutabaga can be a good antifungal if you can take the taste. You can incorporate many of these into your diet once you've started chipping away at the sugar intake to help create a great, effective diet.

The candida diet typically consists of these three things, and if you start to introduce all of these over time, they will help with the candida levels in the body. This is the general outline of what you need, and you can use this in order to help you with your candida condition and make it disappear in a flash.

CHAPTER 4

A Cure For Candida

The only cure for candida is really just resetting the body and making it eat the right things in order to help with the bacteria.

To cure candida, you have to watch what you eat and what you don't eat. You can take all the probiotics and antifungals out there, but if you're not watching what you eat, then you will just reverse your hard work and progress.

This chapter will go over how to cure candida, and how to stop it within its tracks. There are types of foods to eat, and types to avoid. If you're smart about it, you'll be able to really help yourself and your candida condition.

What To Eat

This section will go over eight foods to eat that can help cure candida. You'll be able to eat all of these to help with the overgrowth of the fungus.

The first is vegetables. If you eat plants like kale, Swiss chard, bok choy, and other non-starchy veggies, you'll be able to help reduce the growth of candida while also giving yourself the vitamins and minerals that you need.

They are also rich in folate, which is necessary for those who are sensitive to their candida outgrowth. Ideally, if you're going to eat veggies, make sure you steam or sauté them because it makes it much gentler on the gut.

Clean meats are your next food to eat. Any grass-fed meat, wild-caught fish, or organ meat that is cleaned up would be great for you. They're rich in fat-soluble nutrients, and they will help with the immune system health as well.

This is important because often candida attacks the immune system, but this can also help promote the immune health that is needed for yourself.

Healthy fats are another thing to keep in your arsenal to tackle candida. Various oils such as coconut oil, avocado oil, and even olive oil can be used for gut healing.

These healthy fats are beneficial in many ways, and they can help with the inflammation of the gut. It also has a wealth of various vitamins as well. Coconut oil also contains Caprylic acid, which is proven to help reduce the candida outgrowth.

Cultured foods with bacteria in it such as kimchi, kefir, and sauerkraut are also great to help with a stressed gut. These foods can help to improve the beneficial bacteria levels. You should eat these cultured foods at a moderate level at the beginning because often the candida can flare up from these types of foods since they are pretty strong.

Herbs and spices that heal such as oregano and ginger are also great antibacterial foods. These are good to help get rid of microbes, and in truth, it's an easy thing to ingest. These delicious flavorings can be used in various recipes. They can be put in veggies to give them a kick and even as a supplement if needed. These various herbs and spices are essential to your candida combat, and they're simple to use as well.

Healthy sweeteners such as stevia and xylitol are good if you just need to have sweetener in something like a healthy dessert. They're a better alternative to sugar, which is what you should avoid in the candida diet. Use it sparingly because it can be considered food to some candida cultures.

Tea has also been proven in some cases to help kill off candida. If you're going to drink tea, you should have some black tea because the tannins that are within it have been proven to kill off candida and help with the attack. If you need to calm a flare-up, ideally, ginger teas or any sort of calming teas can help with the gut lining.

Bone broth is an ancient healing food that is making a good comeback in many cases. This is the strongest natural gut medicine for people. Broths can be used as a cleaning method, but it's also a way to help with gut repair.

The collagen within the broth is great for a healthy gut lining. Because it doesn't have sugar, it can help with the reduction of inflammation and also fungal overgrowths too.

What NOT To Eat

Now that we've gone over what you should ideally be consuming on this diet, it's time to talk about what not to eat if you really want to cure candida. These eight foods are the biggest culprits of spreading the pathogen. Often, they are what's holding you back from being fully cured of your candida.

Sugar is your first major cause. Sugar is candida's food, and whether you love it or not, you're going to have to get rid of it. This isn't just the word "sugar" either; this is the whole arsenal of names for sugar such as sucrose, fructose, and other such names.

Obviously, you might not realize it, but a quick google search of the labels that you're reading can tell you whether it's a sugar or not. Often, processed foods and foods that aren't naturally made or sustaining all contain sugar of some shape or form. Therefore, they should be avoided altogether.

Artificial sweeteners are also just as bad, such as aspartame and other such culprits. They are just as responsible for creating a mess with the balance of the gut flora and giving candida the upper hand, so it's best to avoid sugar in any form. You can substitute the need for sugar with various spices as well.

Fruits are typically not bad for you, but they're not good for anyone with candida. The reason for this is because any sugar is considered a good sugar to candida, and they don't help with gut healing. Ideally, severely limiting these the first part of the diet (two weeks) is best.

Once you've eaten a no-sugar or very low-sugar diet, you can introduce some berries or fruits that are low-fructose. You can also eat lemons, grapefruits, and limes as well because they're more citrusy than sugary. Lemon juice is also not bad for you because lemons have antimicrobial characteristics that can help combat candida.

While some such as whole grains are okay, simple grains and processed grains should be avoided. The reason for this is because grains are basically another sugar. They are broken down into carbohydrates, which is basically food for candida. So they should be eaten sparingly or avoided altogether.

Another reason for this is because the gluten within these grains can damage the gut and reverse your progress. You can use some grain-free flours in moderation. Later on, you can use gluten-free grains into your diet, and you can see if they agree with you once you've eliminated a ton of the candida.

Alcohol is something that many of us enjoy to drink, but it's hard on your intestines and can lead to the condition called leaky gut syndrome. Alcohol can also stop the detoxing results, and it can impair some of the pathways that are used in detoxing. Make sure that you don't drink it when you're trying to cleanse.

Dairy in this day and age is basically a junk food because of the antibiotics and hormones that are pushed into it. Often, these cows are fed GMO foods instead of grass, and the dairy that is created is riddled with chemicals like casein that is an extremely sensitive hormone in people with candida.

Along with the casein, many other hormones and chemicals are injected into it, which can do away with some of the progress that you've made.

Ideally, you should make sure that you don't have dairy, except in the cases of kefir and yogurt. Those two should be grass-fed, full-fat, and cultured dairy.

Starchy plants such as various potatoes, beets, and even yams can also be avoided because they feed the candida. If you like legumes such as various beans, lentils, and some nuts, you should also avoid those too because they might cause a food intolerance within you. They're not ideal for your candida cure.

If you do have these, make sure that you wait a bit until most of the candida is healed. Then you can introduce legumes back in to see how your body will take them. If your body can take it, eat them sparingly.

FODMAPs is another food that's often not really pushed. These are the carbs that typically don't get digested by the gut. In some cases, this can be good for you, but for candida, this is bad. They can help feed the candida and other intestinal outgrowths as well if eaten in excess.

Various legumes, some garlic, various onions, apples, and cabbage are part of this. Don't eat these until you start to heal up. See if you can tolerate these before you eat them, then introduce it once again.

Coffee in an excess amount is a major part of irritating the gut. Coffee also can be high in various molds. Topping that with an immune system that is weakened can put a lot of stress on the gut. Some decaf coffees are worse in various cases because of how acidic they are and the amounts of molds that are present within it. If you're going to drink coffee, then make sure that it's organic.

The Cure

With this, you should eat only certain foods and avoid the ones listed. You should keep all sugars out of your body for at least two weeks or as long as a month. Be very minimal and chary of the sugars that you have.

Later on, you can slowly reintroduce some of these foods and see if your body can take it. If it can, you can have it in moderation. All of this should be done in moderation so that you get the best results.

When taking probiotics, take some time to allow your body to get used to them. Often, it does cause a shock to the body, and you might suffer from a few of the symptoms. Often, you'll get a flare-up if you're not careful, so do be chary with it and take it slow before you fully reintroduce it into the body.

The candida cure is really mostly just eating the right foods and avoiding the bad foods. By doing that, you'll slowly eliminate the onslaught that's caused by candida. There really is no other cure, but with the right diet, some probiotics, and the antifungals working together, in three months you can rectify your candida symptoms.

CHAPTER 5

Candida Cure Recipes To Get Started

Now that you know all that you need to know to cure candida, here are a few recipes to get started. It was mentioned in a previous chapter about some of the shakes you can have, and those are just as important as the rest of the diet.

With this, you'll get recipes that work for you, along with some that you can have to help substitute the need for various foods you should stay away from on the candida diet.

Vegetable Broth

This is the first thing to address. Vegetable broth is what you can use on the cleanse, and you should also consider having this when you're cleaning out your gut in general. Vegetable broth is full of a bunch of nutrients, and when the veggies steep within it, the content will be in there as well. This recipe is great and it's tasty as well.

Ingredients:

- 2 chopped onions

- 4 stalks of chopped celery

- 1 t sea salt

- 1 handful of chopped kale

- 3 cloves garlic

- Cayenne pepper to taste

- 2 quarts distilled water

Directions:

1. Take all ingredients and put them together.

2. Boil and then simmer for 20 minutes. Strain out the liquid and remove the veggies. You can have the veggies for later if you want.

3. Drink at least 2-3 bowls of this per day and this recipe should last you two days of the cleanse. You can add some cayenne pepper for spicing and also to increase the anti-inflammatory properties of the broth.

Fiber Bentonite Shake

The fiber bentonite shake will help with improving the digestive flow and takes out many of the various elements of the walls of your gut. It will safely take out any toxins sitting in your intestines.

You can use psyllium husk or acacia powder/pure apple powder for the fiber substitute. Often, psyllium husk can be hard on the gut. You can get some bentonite clay that mixes with water, and it will allow it to go down. You should drink a glass of water immediately after this as well.

Ingredients:

- 1 cup water

- 1 T fiber supplement of choice

- 1 T bentonite clay

Directions:

1. Drink this on an empty stomach, ideally not eating things an hour before. You should try this in the morning, before bedtime, or in the afternoon.

2. Mix it together, drink it, then chase it with water to help push the clay and the fiber supplement. You should drink it at least 2-3 times per day for best results on the cleanse.

The Liver Flush

This is another drink for the cleanse that will help with liver support and protection. This is also good to help flush out toxins in your liver during the candida diet as well.

Ingredients:

- 1 cup water

- 1 clove garlic

- 1 T olive oil

- Chunk of ginger

Directions:

1. Put it all together and blend until smooth texture. You might have to chop it first before blending if your blender isn't good.

2. Drink the Liver Flush water at least 2-3 times a day for best results.

Cinnamon Crisp Cereal

Ingredients:

- 2 cups almond flour
- 2 t cinnamon
- ¼ t baking soda
- ½ t stevia
- 1 egg white
- 1 cup shredded coconut
- ¼ t salt
- ½ t alcohol-free vanilla
- 1 T melted oil
- Blueberries for topping

Directions:

1. Preheat your oven to 350 degrees F. Mix together the flour, cinnamon, baking soda, coconut, and the salt. Set aside.

2. In another bowl, put the vanilla, stevia, and the coconut together. Wait until stevia dissolves.

3. In another bowl, whisk the egg and then put it within the liquid mixture and whisk again.

4. Put the liquid ingredients with the dry ingredients and then make a dough. Put it on a piece of parchment paper and then place on a baking sheet. Bake it for 12 minutes

5. Once done, cut the dough into strips and then set it aside, creating small squares.

6. Cool it, then serve with coconut or almond milk.

Apple Yogurt Parfait With Walnuts

Ingredients:

- 1 apple
- 1 cup yogurt
- Handful walnuts
- Cinnamon for topping

Directions:

1. Chop the ingredients and then do the apples on bottom, then yogurt, then walnuts, alternating.

2. Put cinnamon on top to serve.

Buckwheat Ravioli

Ingredients (For Filling):

- 1 T olive oil

- 1 clove minced garlic

- ½ pound various greens

- Salt and pepper to taste

- ½ cup chopped onion

- 1 pound ground meat

- ¼ t nutmeg

Ravioli:

- 2 cups buckwheat flour

- 2 egg yolks

- 1 T olive oil

- ¼ t salt

- 1 egg

Directions:

1. When making the filling, preheat the oil, and then put in the onion and garlic. Cook for about 4 minutes.

2. Add in the meat and then cook for another five minutes. Add in the greens, nutmeg, and spices to taste, cooking for about 2 minutes.

3. For the filling, mix the buckwheat flour and salt together and then put a well at the center. Add in the rest of the ingredients.

4. Beat the mixture in a gentle manner without incorporating the flour. Mix it together until the dough is too stiff to mix with your fork.

5. Now, take half the dough at a time and roll it out to about 1/8 an inch thick, then cut out three circles. You can then put a tablespoon of the filling into the center and put a bit of water on the edges.

6. Put another dough circle on top and then press it until it's a sealed ravioli. Put it into a flour surface and continue process with the rest of the circles and filling.

7. Bring 2 quarts of water to the boiling point, and then pour in the ravioli, cooking for about 5-7 minutes until tender.

8. Remove, and then serve it immediately.

Chicken Picatta

Ingredients:

- 1 pound of chicken tenders
- 4 T olive oil
- 1 clove minced garlic
- 1 t coconut flour
- 2 T lemon juice
- 2 T chopped parsley
- Salt and pepper to taste
- ¼ cup minced onion
- 2 cups chicken stock
- 1 T butter
- ¼ cup green olives
- Slices of lemon to garnish

Directions:

1. Preheat oven to 250. Put the chicken tenders onto wax paper and then pound until ¼ inch thick.

2. Liberally sprinkle with salt and pepper, turning each one over and seasoning well. Place on a plate on the counter.

3. Put the chicken tenders in a skillet and then cook for 1-2 minutes or until browned. Continue until they're all done.

4. Once that's done, add in the onions and the garlic then sauté for at least a minute.

5. Add in the broth and the flour and then simmer for about 3 minutes. Take the skillet off the heat and put the rest of the ingredients together to combine.

6. Put the chicken tenders on a serving plate and then put the sauce over it, adding parsley and lemon to garnish.

7. Until it's time to combine the chicken and sauce together, you should keep them in an oven to keep them warm.

Sesame Cauliflower Rounds

Ingredients:

- 4 cups cauliflower florets, chopped in a rough manner
- 2 T chia seeds
- 1 t salt
- ½ cup water
- ¼ cup golden flaxseed meal
- ½ cup sesame seeds
- 3 T melted coconut oil
- 1 cup sesame seeds for topping

Directions:

1. Put the cauliflower in a food processor and then process it until it's the size of rice.

2. Put together the flaxseed, seeds, salt, water, and the coconut oil. Let it become a dough.

3. Chill it for about 3-4 hours.

4. Preheat the oven, and then put the dough into balls and then roll them into the sesame seeds.

5. Place them between two sheets of parchment paper and flatten them to about 2-3 inches round.

6. Continue this, and then bake it for 30 minutes on each side, cooling before serving.

These are recipes to get you started with your candida diet. They are candida friendly and you'll be able to use these to help not only with a cleanse, but the diet will bring you back to snuff as well.

Conclusion

Thank you again for taking the time to learn about how to combat candida.

I hope you realized that this diet is the way to reverse the effects of candida. There is no other cure, and in truth, your diet is what will affect candida, whether it be for good or for bad.

Don't let your diet continue to hold you back and start to take the time to really improve your life through the use of the candida diet. You owe it to yourself to really rectify the situations you're put in, and candida can be fixed with just a few diet changes as well.

With that being said, it's time to move onto the next step. Your next step is simple, and that is to start taking the time to really work on your candida diet.

In truth, it will take a couple of doctor visits, but if you know you have it, speak with your doctor confidentially. Your doctor can help you get started, and you can take control of your candida before it controls you.

Did You Enjoy This Book?

I want to thank you for purchasing and reading this book. I really hope you got a lot out of it.

Can I ask a quick favor?

If you enjoyed this book, I would really appreciate it if you could leave me a positive review on Amazon.

I love getting feedback from my customers, and reviews on Amazon really do make a difference. I read all my reviews and would really appreciate your thoughts.

Thanks so much.

NATALIE PETERSON

Made in the
USA
Monee, IL